Easiest Way To Get Rid Of Pregnancy Hemorrhoids In 2024

Your Essential Handbook For Overcoming Pregnancy Hemorrhoids With Confidence

By Kimberley Garcia

Copyright

Disclaimer

Please note that the material contained in this book, titled "Easiest Way to Get Rid of Pregnancy Haemorrhoids in 2024," is intended solely to provide basic information. This information is not meant to serve as a replacement for the diagnosis or treatment provided by a qualified medical expert. If you have any inquiries concerning a medical problem, you should always consult with your primary care physician or another trained health expert.

The author and publisher of this book do not make any claims or warranties of any kind, whether they are stated or implied, regarding the completeness, accuracy, reliability, appropriateness, or availability of the information that is provided within these pages. Therefore, any reliance that you place on such material is entirely the result of your risk.

The material in this book is based on general knowledge as of the date of release (2024), and the author and publisher do not accept any responsibility for errors, inaccuracies, or omissions. The reader is recommended to validate the information supplied with additional sources and to see a healthcare expert for specialized advice tailored to their unique circumstances.

The author and publisher disclaim all liability for any loss, injury, or damage experienced as a direct or indirect consequence of the use or application of any material contained in this book. Readers should use their discretion and judgment, taking into consideration their specific circumstances, when applying the material offered in this book.

About The Author

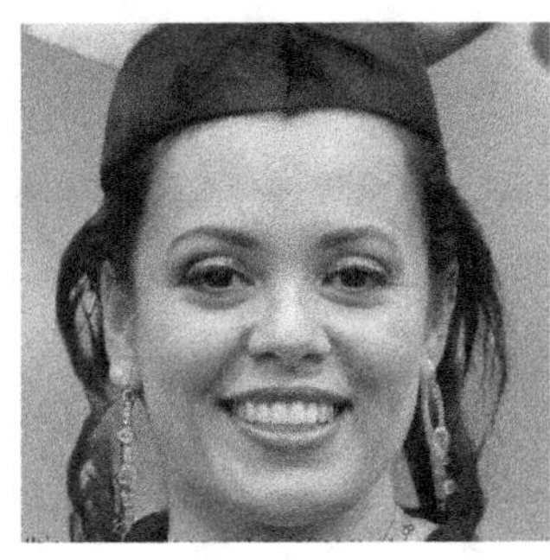 Kimberley Garcia is the brilliant and caring voice behind "Easiest Way To Get Rid Of Pregnancy Hemorrhoids In 2024." As a devoted medical practitioner, Kimberley combines her knowledge and extensive understanding of healthcare to provide vital insights into an issue that impacts many pregnant moms.

Kimberley Garcia has dedicated her professional life to promoting the well-being of her patients. Her love for women's health, particularly throughout the transforming journey of pregnancy, has prompted her to offer her knowledge and practical guidance in this thorough handbook.

Beyond her position as a healthcare practitioner, Kimberley is a loving spouse, navigating the challenges of married life with a commitment to health, happiness, and mutual support. This personal part of her life provides a human touch to her work, as she knows the complexity of combining personal and professional duties.

In "Easiest Way To Get Rid Of Pregnancy Hemorrhoids In 2024," Kimberley Garcia combines her medical experience with empathy and compassion, seeking to equip readers with the skills they need to handle the issues of pregnant hemorrhoids. Her commitment to giving factual, dependable, and accessible information shows through in every chapter, making this book a wonderful resource for pregnant moms seeking comfort and solace.

With a genuine desire to make a good impact on the lives of her readers, Kimberley welcomes you to join her on this journey of information, support, and empowerment as you begin on the path to a more pleasant and pleasurable pregnancy.

Table Of Contents

INTRODUCTION

Welcome to "Easiest Way To Get Rid Of Pregnancy Hemorrhoids In 2024." Pregnancy is a magnificent and transforming adventure, but it also comes with its particular set of obstacles. One such problem that many pregnant women confront is the discomfort and anguish associated with pregnancy hemorrhoids. As we venture into the year 2024, our awareness of this widespread yet frequently neglected ailment has improved, bringing forth creative and effective treatments for alleviation.

In this thorough book, we traverse the complicated environment of pregnant hemorrhoids, bringing you insights, practical guidance, and the latest ways to reduce your agony. Whether you're a soon-to-be parent seeking precautionary measures, presently battling with symptoms, or looking for the fastest ways to find relief, this book is your trusted guide on the route to a more comfortable and pleasurable pregnancy.

For those wanting quick relief, our examination of the fastest methods to get rid of pregnant hemorrhoids in 2024 contains a range of choices, from over-the-counter therapies to prescription drugs and calming home cures. The emphasis is not just on fast resolution but also on encouraging long-term well-being.

Pregnant individuals often experience hemorrhoids, which are swollen veins around the anus that can be uncomfortable and painful. These can be attributed to normal bodily changes during pregnancy, such as increased blood volume, an expanding uterus, and changing hormone levels. The duration of pregnancy hemorrhoids can vary, lasting for days, weeks, months, or even longer. It is important not to suffer in silence and to focus on reducing and coping with hemorrhoids, as they may not go away until after delivery. There are tips and tricks available to help relieve pregnancy hemorrhoids.

What Are Pregnancy Hemorrhoids?

Hemorrhoids are itchy, inflamed varicose veins in and around the anus. They're common in pregnancy, and they can be pretty uncomfortable for the person experiencing them.

Causes of Hemorrhoids During Pregnancy

Hemorrhoids are frequent during pregnancy, due to impaired blood flow and blood vessels that expand because of higher-than-usual blood volume. That additional blood can cause hemorrhoids to plump up to the size of a marble, and your enlarging uterus also places greater pressure on the pelvic veins, aggravating the swelling.

Prolonged sitting, weight increase, restricted physical activity, low-fiber diets, constipation, and the natural hormonal changes that occur during pregnancy can all contribute to developing hemorrhoids. Additionally, the strain required in delivering delivery vaginally might induce hemorrhoids.

One study indicated that of about 40% of the pregnant individuals surveyed who acquired hemorrhoids, 60% got them in the third trimester, and around 34% developed hemorrhoids in the postpartum period. The others got them early in pregnancy. Some patients also developed anal fissures.

Anal fissures, which are tiny rips in the lining of the anus, sometimes occur in tandem with constipation and hemorrhoids. These microscopic incisions normally heal on their own over a few weeks, and they can be fairly unpleasant, making bowel motions more uncomfortable and personal hygiene more complex.

How to Prevent Hemorrhoids During Pregnancy

The easiest method to deal with hemorrhoids is to avoid developing them in the first place. You may apply various effective measures to prevent them. This includes preventing constipation (which aggravates hemorrhoids) by ingesting lots of fluids, eating a high-fiber diet, and exercising frequently.

Not straining on the toilet when having a bowel movement might also assist in preventing hemorrhoids. However, even after following this advice, hemorrhoids can still develop—especially during pregnancy.

Symptoms of Pregnancy Hemorrhoids

The symptoms of hemorrhoids could include the following:

- Pain in the anus, especially with bowel movements
- Blood on the toilet paper, covering the feces, or in the toilet
- Itchy anal canal
- Burning or swelling
- Tender lump at the anus (for external hemorrhoids)

The Fastest Way to Get Rid of Hemorrhoids During Pregnancy

Pregnant women often develop hemorrhoids, which are painful and itchy swollen veins in or around the anus. These varicose veins are caused by poor blood flow. Hemorrhoids tend to worsen immediately after giving birth, but gradually improve during the postpartum period.

While you may not be able to get rid of hemorrhoids in pregnancy entirely, the following ways may lessen the pain associated with them. Making efforts to lessen the discomfort of hemorrhoids can also lower the size of these bulging veins, and eventually help them go away.

Take a Sitz Bath

For those asking how to rapidly obtain treatment for pregnant hemorrhoids at home, a warm-water soak could reduce discomfort. That doesn't mean you have to fill a whole bathtub; instead, you may buy a tiny plastic tub (called a "sitz bath") from the drugstore.

Fill it with warm water and set it over your toilet. Sit in it for 15 minutes, many times a day—especially after having a bowel movement. To get the most out of your sitz bath, try these tips:

- Add extra water to keep the temperature pleasant.
- Try an over-the-counter sitz bath with baking soda (sodium bicarbonate), but avoid aromatic kinds if you are sensitive.
- Try 1/2 cup Epsom salt per gallon of warm water for relief.
- Don't stand too fast when you're finished; go nice and leisurely.
- Gently pat yourself dry with a clean towel before getting dressed.

Apply Ice

Try alternating ice packs with warm-water soaks. Apply the ice for 15 minutes at a time to minimize swelling. However, you shouldn't lay ice directly on the hemorrhoids; always use a washcloth or other barrier.

Try Witch Hazel Pads

Some women try curing hemorrhoids with witch hazel. You may buy witch hazel pads in supermarkets and use them to wipe after going to the restroom.

Witch hazel is an astringent, which means that it can help temporarily decrease hemorrhoids by sucking away water from the tissue. You may use a liquid type of witch hazel to administer a cold compress or try presoaked witch hazel pads to help alleviate itching, soreness, and swelling.

For extra comfort, chill the witch hazel in the fridge before applying it to hemorrhoids.

Use Soft, Wet Toilet Paper

Using unscented, white toilet tissue can minimize irritation, and it could help to dampen the cloth before you wipe around your anus. You may also buy specifically medicated moist towelettes to use instead of toilet tissue. Avoid wipes with strong chemicals or powerful perfumes, as they may cause sensitivities.

Implement Lifestyle Changes

Some of the most robust and efficient therapies to get rid of hemorrhoids during pregnancy may be found in simple lifestyle adjustments. These same measures can also prevent hemorrhoids in the first place. Taking care of your health—including how you exercise, eat, and rest—makes hemorrhoids less of a pain in the derrière.

Try these ways to cure your hemorrhoids:
- Avoid straining on the toilet.
- Eat meals high in fiber.
- Take stool softeners (with your doctor's clearance).
- Drink at least six to eight glasses of water a day.
- Avoid sitting or standing for lengthy periods of time.

- Lie on your left side when sleeping or watching TV.
- Avoid lifting hefty weights.

Ask About Topical Anesthetics Or Medicated Suppositories

If the discomfort or itching becomes excessive, ask your practitioner to prescribe a topical anesthetic or a safe medicated suppository.

The best treatment for hemorrhoids may be a stool softener, as it reduces constipation and straining that can worsen irritation. Speak with your healthcare professional before using a laxative or stool stimulant while pregnant.

Do Hemorrhoids Go Away On Their Own?

Unlike persistent hemorrhoids, pregnancy-related episodes are nearly always transitory and should go away once your baby is delivered. If your hemorrhoids continue, talk to your doctor about a new treatment approach.

When to Contact Your Health Care Provider

If you have hemorrhoids or you fear you might, let your healthcare provider know at your next prenatal appointment. Don't hesitate to call their office if you have any questions or concerns between appointments.

Your medical professional can help you design a treatment plan. If your hemorrhoids are really painful, becoming worse, or making going to the bathroom problematic, check in with your doctor immediately.

Conclusion

As we end "Easiest Way To Get Rid Of Pregnancy Hemorrhoids In 2024," I want to offer my thanks for allowing me to be a part of your path toward a more pleasant and happy pregnancy. Navigating the obstacles of pregnant hemorrhoids is no minor effort, and your commitment to obtaining knowledge and treatment is laudable.

Throughout this book, we've studied the subtleties of pregnant hemorrhoids - from understanding their nature and causes to proactive preventative methods, symptom assessment, and the fastest strategies to get relief. It has been my honest desire to present you with a thorough and sensitive resource, that integrates medical knowledge with practical guidance and real-life anecdotes.

Remember, your well-being is of the utmost importance, and taking proactive actions to control pregnant hemorrhoids is a witness to your commitment to a healthy and happy pregnancy. Whether you're just starting your journey, presently battling with symptoms, or seeking postpartum treatment, the information offered here is aimed at helping you through each step.

As you move forward, consider this book not just as a source of knowledge but as a companion on your road to comfort and confidence. Embrace holistic ideas, gain strength from personal experiences, and apply practical advice to your daily life. Your road toward a hemorrhoid-free pregnancy is a tribute to your tenacity and dedication.

In conclusion, I encourage you to emphasize self-care, seek help when required, and embrace the challenges of pregnancy with the assurance that you are not alone. Congratulations on taking the initiative to invest in your well-being and the well-being of your developing family.

I wish you a wonderful and easy pregnancy journey and a future filled with health, pleasure, and the many delights of motherhood.

With warmth and best wishes,

Kimberley Garcia

I HAVE A REQUEST

Dear **Reader**,

I hope this message finds you well. I am writing to kindly request your feedback and review of my recently published book, **"Easiest Way To Get Rid Of Pregnancy Hemorrhoids In 2024."** Your thoughts and opinions are incredibly important to me, and I would greatly appreciate your honest review.

Your review will not only provide valuable insights but also help other potential readers make informed decisions about whether to explore the book. As a fellow reader, your perspective is highly regarded.

Here's how you can help:

- *Read the Book*: If you haven't already had the chance to read **"Easiest Way To Get Rid Of Pregnancy Hemorrhoids In 2024,"** I'd be happy to provide you with a complimentary copy in your preferred format (eBook or paperback).

- *Share Your Review*: After reading the book, please take a moment to share your thoughts by leaving a review on popular book retail platforms, such as Amazon, Goodreads, or any other platform where you prefer to review books.
- *Be Honest and Constructive*: Your honest opinion is what matters most. Whether you loved the book or had some critical feedback, I welcome your insights. Constructive criticism is just as valuable as praise.
- *Spread the Word*: If you found the book enjoyable and enlightening, consider sharing your review with your friends and family or on your social media platforms to help others discover it.

Your support in providing a review will not only be deeply appreciated but will also be instrumental in spreading the message and impact of the book. Your input will guide future readers and play a vital role in its success.

Thank you for taking the time to consider my request. Your support means a great deal to me, and I am grateful for your willingness to share your thoughts on the **"Easiest Way To Get Rid Of Pregnancy Hemorrhoids In 2024."**

I wish you an enriching reading experience, and I look forward to hearing from you.

Warm regards,

Kimberley Garcia

ADDITIONAL RESOURCES

Dear Reader, I am here again:

Thank you for your support and interest in **"Easiest Way To Get Rid Of Pregnancy Hemorrhoids In 2024."** If you enjoyed this book and are looking for more valuable resources and engaging content, I would recommend some of my books that you might find intriguing:

1. **"Best Parenting Book For Kids With ADHD"**: *An ADHD Parenting Guide for Raising Hyperactive Kids, Dealing with Behavioral Issues, and Supporting Explosive Children*
2. **"Finding Relief"**: *10 Home Remedies To Relieve Menstrual Cramps*
3. **"Successful Parenting Of Kids With Autism"**: *Easy Steps To Raising Brilliant Autistic Kids*
4. **"Single Mom's Pregnancy Guide"**: *A Comprehensive Guide For Single Mothers*
5. **"Pregnancy Cookbook With Nutritional Information"**: *The Complete Healthy Guide To Optimal Prenatal Nutrition And Real Food*

For Pregnancy With 30+ Recipes For Your Pregnancy Meal Plan

6. **"The Complete Guide For Trending Baby Names In 2024"**: *A Thoughtful Up-To-Date Guide To Selecting Unique And Timeless Baby Names For Expecting Mothers, Fathers And Parents*

To explore these books, please visit my Author Central Page on Amazon. **You can scan the QR code below or click the link to visit my Author Central:**

https://www.amazon.com/author/kimberley_garcia

Your continued support means the world to me, and I am committed to providing you with valuable information and inspiration on your journey as a woman.

Thank you for being a part of this community, and I hope my books continue to bring you joy and empowerment.

Warm regards,
Kimberley Garcia

PS: *Don't forget to check out my Author Central page on Amazon to discover more of my books. Your feedback and reviews are always appreciated!*